I0477241

What's so Good about Feelin' Good?

What's so Good about Feelin' Good?

Making Sense of the Nonsense

Zaib Bey

Copyright © 2010 by Zaib Bey.

Library of Congress Control Number: 2010903317
ISBN: Hardcover   978-1-4500-6011-0
               Softcover   978-1-4500-6010-3

All rights reserved. No part of this book may be reproduced or transmitted in any form or by any means, electronic or mechanical, including photocopying, recording, or by any information storage and retrieval system, without permission in writing from the copyright owner.

Zaib Bey/087-52-1435
Center for Common Sense Self-Help © 2008 by Zaib Bey
PO Box 5467
Kaneohe, Hawaii 96744
Phone: 808/372-2577
E-mail: zzaib@yahoo.com

This book was printed in the United States of America.

To order additional copies of this book, contact:
Xlibris Corporation
1-888-795-4274
www.Xlibris.com
Orders@Xlibris.com
61681

CONTENTS

Prologue 7

Introduction 9

Chapter I. A Few Facts about Drugs 13

Chapter II. In Search of Happiness 17

Chapter III. Feelin' Good 19

Chapter IV. Choice 22

Chapter V. Making Sense of Your World 25

Chapter VI. A Language That Makes Sense 28

Chapter VII. More About Feelin' Good 33

Chapter VIII. Understanding Feelings 36

Chapter IX. Clearing-up Mental Confusion 41

Chapter X. The Common Sense Perspective of Needs 48

Chapter XI. Compulsion-Driven Behaviors/

The Nature of Addiction 55

Self-Test Answers 57

Index 61

PROLOGUE

Creative design provides the feelings associated with pleasure as the reward for survival and pain and discomfort (dis-ease), as the punishment for behaviors that conflict with the supreme dictate to survive. Of all the species that populate the planet, man alone has created work and convinced his fellow man that pleasure in the absence of work was a sin.

Though both Earth and man have been innately endowed with all the resources necessary to sustain themselves, only man has chosen to disrupt this order. It appears that only man has been endowed with the power to intervene in this natural order, and it also appears that man has even determined himself justified to place himself ahead of Mother Nature, forgetting the prime edict, all the time knowing "it's not nice to mess with Mother Nature." Maybe we should be more aware of what we are bringing upon ourselves.

INTRODUCTION

It is generally accepted that "the pursuit of happiness" is an "inalienable right" of all people. This right (the right to pursue) is guaranteed by the Constitution of the United States, and most of its citizens are actively engaged in the daily pursuit of it. And happiness is only one of the many pots of gold perceived at the end of these rainbows.

To the best of my knowledge, there exists no standard or tool sufficient to quantifiably measure this quality we refer to as "happiness," and the sciences tell us "if you can't measure it, it doesn't exist." Since there exists no empirically proven or verifiable entity as "happiness," the elusive search for an effective technique for achieving "happiness" would appear to be an exercise in futility.

The fact is, in the real world, there are times when, in spite of our best efforts, we just can't seem to find that illusive "happy place." It is, therefore, reasonable to assume that the resulting state of dis-ease (emotional turmoil) we all experience at some time or another in our lives will be a product of any one of at least three of the currently popular paradigms, which suggests that most physically and emotionally unhealthy conditions may be attributed to factors such as:

1. Genetic imbalance—inherited traits
2. Social stressors—the wife, the family, the dog, the devil
3. Environmental stressors—gender issues, the job, racism, sexism, health.

   These are only a few of the major challenges that regularly impact the individual's emotional/feeling state.

The result? Many find themselves resorting to compulsion-driven behaviors, which may include abuse of alcohol and other substances as mechanisms to relieve or cope with the simple act of daily living. Some, unable to cope, find themselves voluntarily seeking help from mental health professionals, while others may involuntarily end up institutionalized.

In the case of drugs, one may reasonably argue that, as the level of drug consumption increases, the effects may create the illusion that the problems of their world exist outside of their control. As a result, many will view their life situation as hopeless and themselves as helpless/powerless. Often, the prevailing paradigms appear to perpetuate this illusion: "Admit that my life has become unmanageable and that I am powerless." The result is fairly predictable; many of those suffering/experiencing dis-ease continue to seek their salvation from substances with potentials for abuse or other compulsion-driven behaviors that appear to offer an external solution to the problems of their daily life. Unfettered, these are the cases that will likely end up in institutions that provide mental illness/substance abuse (MISA) services.

MAKING SENSE OF BEHAVIOR

The need to understand behavior is probably one of humankind's greatest desires, second only to the need/desire to make sense of behaviors. It appears the two concepts are not necessarily synonymous.

So what is behavior?

Though we spend much time labeling the sundry ways specific actions may manifest (categorizing all under the rubric "behavior"), little time has truly been spent developing a clear definition of what it ("behavior") is exactly.

I was recently discussing the term *compulsion* with a client and was caught off guard when he asked, "What's the difference between a compulsion and a habit?" The dialogue continued with a clarification of the term *compulsion*. My definition was as follows: *compulsion*. the drive to perform a behavior for which there is an anticipated payoff. The payoff, most often, manifests as a neurochemical rush that we humans generally interpret or describe as "good feelin's." There followed a description of how memory activates the system that stimulates behavior and points out how it (memory) is generally characterized, based upon recall of the ultimate payoff for the behavior, that is, was it positive or negative? Of course, there will always be the follow-up question (the one rarely asked): Is it still paying off?

At the compulsive level, the behavior appears to be no longer cognitively driven but merely habitual responses that continue to manifest even in the absence of the anticipated/identifiable payoff. The script generally sounds something like this:

"I used to . . ."

"But now I only . . ."

"And for some unknown reason, I just continue to . . ."

In short, what at some point in time seemed to make "perfect sense," for some reason, now makes "no sense" at all, yet the compulsive nature of the behavior continues to drive you on. You just don't seem able to stop. The key words here are *seem* and *able.*

Of course, you can stop! You only need to give yourself a good-enough reason/payoff to make the decision to stop and then develop a replacement behavior sufficiently rewarding that you may be reasonably assured that you will use it in future circumstances to replace the old behavior. Remember, no one develops or changes a behavior for no reason at all.

CHAPTER ONE

A Few Facts about Drugs

Historically, large numbers of people in our society indulge in some form of compulsive / compulsion-driven behavior and / or use some form of drug (as prescribed or in other ways), and by adulthood, most have engaged in some form of alcohol or drug consumption. In the case of alcohol, the National Institute on Alcohol Abuse and Alcoholism (NIAAA), in 2001, has gone so far as to set what it considers "safe limits" of consumption: fourteen drinks per week for men and no more than seven drinks per week for women. Updated, NIAAA recommends "no more than one drink per day for men and women older than sixty-five years."

This finding has been supported by a report from the American Heart Association saying that "drinking moderate amounts of alcohol can serve as [protection] against coronary heart disease (CHD)." This report is cited from the *New England Journal of Medicine* 1993, 329, 1829-1834, and though it may be in conflict with many other reports by this same organization, more than a dozen prospective studies support its contention that there exists "a consistent, strong, dose-response relation between increasing alcohol consumption and decreasing incidence of CHD." The data are similar across gender and geographic and ethnic groups, and the conclusions consistently suggest that consumption of one or two drinks per day is associated with a reduction in risk of CHD of approximately 30 percent to 50 percent." This finding should not obscure the fact that differing tolerance levels will likely skewer the data.

This writing simply contends that, in the future, we must begin to accept that abusive forms of behavior, which includes consumption/use of alcohol or other drugs, are compulsion-driven products of the mind (internally driven) and should be given at least equal consideration as those other external factors most usually considered as the source of problem behaviors that may result from the use of alcohol or other drugs.

For this writing, I will attempt to restrain myself to a discussion of compulsions associated with the abusive use of alcohol and other addictive drugs (AOAD).

Little that follows may be considered new. It is anticipated that, as a result of this reading, you will become reconnected to knowledge you may simply have lost touch with.

An abstract from *Military Psychology* (1992), vol. 4, no. 4, pages 191-205, cites the "use of stimulants to ameliorate the effects of sleep loss during sustained performance." The article by Harvey Babkoff and Gerald P. Krueger discusses the military's uses of and continued experiments into the impact of stimulant drugs on "performance due to sleep loss and sustained operations." In an abstract from the *International Journal of Aviation Psychology* (1996), vol. 6, no. 4, pages 379-397, titled "Methamphetamine Effects on Cognitive Processing During Extended Wakefulness," Douglas A. Weigmann, Robert R. Stanny, et al., conclude that "amphetamine treatments decreased subjective sleepiness during the night and tended to increase subjective sleep latencies during a post-testing sleep period."

Historically, drugs have been used to sustain performance (during military ground and air operations) over long periods of time or to offset the effects of sleep deprivation on sustained performance. The results of such studies continue to be reviewed and their results evaluated for future theoretical and practical applications. It is hypocritical to even attempt to overlook the fact that drug use, in its varied forms, continues to play important roles in many aspects of our daily lives. From school to professional athletic performance, issues of legitimacy and legality may create more problems than they resolve.

Leileilani (a made-up name) is a single mother of three children ages six, eight, and eleven. She is a working professional nurse, maintains a second job as a bartender six nights a week, and provides care to an elderly couple on weekends. She is attractive, well respected, and accepted in her community. Somehow she also seems able to find time to maintain a personal relationship and to care for her home and children.

Leileilani was introduced to methamphetamine (ice) by her boyfriend approximately three years ago and bluntly admits she does not know how she could sustain her multifaceted regimen without help. On several occasions, she has attempted to "cut back." She says it's "too difficult," and she is having difficulties coming to grips with the fact that she has become dependent on the substance. She is currently seeking help and believes she may be more successful this time since the children are beginning to assume some of the responsibilities of the home and are more independent. However, she still is unsure how she will cope with the work schedule. She needs the additional funds to sustain her family's standard of living. She is also toying with the idea of giving up her relationship as he continues to use and is not likely to change his behaviors.

Do we conclude that her use of methamphetamine is less legitimate than that of the soldier, airman, truck driver, or commercial pilot? Are sport promoters, owners, and management aware of the extent some are willing to go to attain and maintain the huge monetary benefits that push some to play through pain and, in many cases, shorten their careers to enhance their "bottom-line" attendance numbers? Will the elimination of performance-enhancing drugs (PEDs) detract from the attendance at professional as well as amateur sporting events? Is the real issue the use or the potential negative impact of use on individuals, families, and society in general (when use evolves into addiction/ chemical dependence)?

The simple facts are chemical dependence, most commonly referred to as addiction, is not the goal sought in any of the above cited cases. When queried, individuals will most often suggest "it [the issues associated with chemical dependency] just seems to happen. Things were working out just fine, and all of a sudden . . ."

The uninformed constantly find themselves asking (with all the available negative data), why do people continue to do drugs?

The answer is so obvious. It's baffling, to the informed, that anyone could ask such a question. The answer is what we all know and has been consistently validated by research: *drugs work.*

Let's not delude ourselves. In many cases intellectually and physically, drugs may provide the competitive edge. Innumerable college students may share how they were able to stay focused (maintain the edge) after many nights of staying awake, studying, and preparing for exams. The real world fact is, both physically and emotionally, drugs make unbearable situations bearable, and in many cases, are like the American credit card system: though you're up to your ears in debt, even though you don't have a dime in the bank, you can still feel good about the fact that you're living in a home that neither you or your inheritors will ever own, driving a car that will be too old to have value by the time it is paid off, submitting yourself to personal surgical processes that will enhance your outward appearance, and ultimately, though you may like what you see in the mirror and others will marvel at your lifestyle, in the end, you will not have improved the quality of your life one iota.

CHAPTER TWO

In Search of Happiness

The problem? Very few of those persons seeking happiness are able to clearly articulate what it will consist of once found, but all tend to agree, "it will feel good!" Having no objective view of what this illusive "happiness" is, few are able to offer a proven, effective technique for achieving it. More important, rarely is the individual able to offer an operational definition for what this elusive "happiness" will "feel like," if they were able to achieve it, but most are absolutely certain they will know it when they feel it, and once experienced, the search begins to feel or experience a more intense sense of happiness.

Some, unable to find that "good feeling" others appear to be experiencing, develop defense mechanisms to ward off the discomfort associated with situations they find themselves unable to cope with. For many, seeking that illusive "feel good" sensation, alcohol and other substances with potential for abuse are often adopted as mechanisms to achieve this "feel good" state, relieve general discomfort, or simply cope with daily chores of living. Many, still unable to cope, find themselves voluntarily seeking help from mental health professionals, while others often, involuntarily, end up institutionalized.

As the prevailing authorities tend to perpetuate this illusion, those suffering from illnesses that may be psychological, drug related, or both mental illness and substance abuse (MISA), more commonly referred to as "the dually diagnosed," tend to seek their salvation, more and more, from substances with potentials for abuse or other resources (to include support groups) that offer external solutions to the problems of their daily life. Unfettered and unhelped, these are the cases that will likely end up in institutions that provide MISA services.

An honest look at most societies will reveal that historically, a majority of the world's populations indulge in some form of compulsive/compulsion-driven behavior. An even closer look will probably show that by adulthood, most will have engaged in some form of alcohol or drug consumption (legal or prescribed). Where in Western societies consumption of alcohol has been accepted as a part of the socially acceptable rituals of daily living, in Central American and Eastern cultures, other forms have been incorporated into the daily rituals associated with living. These rituals take on many forms (running, reading, sex, support-group meetings). In fact, the form is immaterial; the significance is solely related to the need/desire to seek the comfort one has been unable to access internally from some external resource, and humankind has proven extraordinarily resourceful in accomplishing this task.

Since the behaviors associated with the terms compulsion/ addiction are so numerous, for this writing, I will restrain myself to a discussion of the compulsions associated with the abusive use of alcohol and other addictive drugs (AOAD).

CHAPTER THREE

Feelin' Good

Over the years, Alcohol and Other Drugs (AOD) have become an acceptable solution to the resolution of pain or discomfort and that is primarily why abuse of drugs (legal or illegal) is currently viewed as one of the major problems affecting most world cultures.

The form of thinking which triggers the compulsive use of drugs suggests to the individual that negative aspects of their world are going to change, simply because they feel better or good or are able to remove themselves from the inconvenience of any feelings at all. We have become a nation of feelers, but we don't like to experience uncomfortable feelings, much less pain. For this reason, as a society, we begin, as early as infancy, the administration of drugs (in varying forms); to eliminate pain; to help us feel better or to simply *Not Feel At All.*

The fact is the human genome is innately predisposed to seek pleasure.

According to noted neurologist Antonio Damasio (2003), "Feelings of pain or pleasure or some quality in between are the bedrock of our minds."

We are "wired to seek pleasure," and this pleasure-seeking propensity appears to be innate. This feeling of pleasure we all seem to be in search of appears to be the natural reward the brain provides for engaging in behaviors that sustain life, i.e., the species.[1] It therefore makes sense that we humans would be equally predisposed to avoid experiencing pain or even discomfort (punishment for engaging in behaviors detrimental to our survival). We also learn very early in life that there is a pill or potion that will help us to achieve any of these feeling or nonfeeling states instantly at will.

The good news (that every drug user is aware of and those casual consumers of aspirin, diet pills, cough medicines, etc., who consider themselves nonconsumers, choose not to acknowledge) is, once again, *drugs work.*

The bad news is many of these substances, both legal and illegal, have properties that may result in "chemical dependence" or addiction as it is most commonly labeled.

The obvious question here is, Can we feel better without drugs?

And the answer is, of course, you can, but it requires the activation of those natural chemical elements that the brain provides as a reward for having accomplished something deserving the reward/experience of pleasure. And this requires activity of some sort. Be it the initiation of a relaxation exercise or some physical activity, there is effort involved. Only through the use of stimulant drugs, alcohol, or tranquilizers can one experience or not experience the emotional or physical aspects of their daily life without activity of some sort.

Unfortunately, as previously stated, the properties that constitute most stimulant drugs, alcohol, or tranquilizers, have the potential to eventually negatively impact the brain's ability to naturally produce those chemicals that result in the same feeling state. The sense of well-being or euphoria the body/mind seeks

---

1. In fact, absence of the ability to experience or reflect pleasure has been established as a prime indicator/symptom of children experiencing autistic syndrome disorders (ASDs). Though there appears to be little evidenced-based research in this area, I am sure this correlation will be established, at some point in the near future.

may become dependent upon these outside resources to ease the resulting state of dis-ease. The end product is predictable; the consumer becomes convinced that they can only attain this sense of calm or well-being we in the helping profession refer to as homeostasis (natural state of calm) by indulging in compulsive/ habitual behaviors, which may manifest as gambling, drug use, Pac Man, Free Cell, etc. Regardless of the vehicle one takes to feel good, the obvious follow-on would be curiosity as to how much to feel better and better and better, and you say you wonder how one might get "hooked."

For the consumer, the really good news is you do not have to become dependent on drugs or engage in other abhorrent behaviors to enjoy these good feelings or to attain a sense of well-being. You can learn to experience the feeling or the emotions you desire without alcohol/drugs or engaging in other compulsion-driven behaviors.

CHAPTER FOUR

Choice

It appears that every living organism on this planet is, from conception, is genetically coded to sustain and to regenerate itself. Uniquely, only the human genome appears to have developed the capacity to modify, at will, its innate tendencies, and we commonly recognize this as "free will" or more commonly "choice." Though we are programmed to survive, the quality of life/living is a product of choice.

For over twenty-five years, I have listened to supposedly mature adults use childlike logic to explain away the errors (poor choices) they make in their daily lives. In hindsight, it's truly baffling to hear otherwise intelligent people make statements such as "I really should have . . ."

The look on their faces when I respond emphatically, "No, you should not have!" is one of utter dismay. Of course, I quickly follow up with a rehash of the first lesson I give to all my consumers, i.e., everything in life is exactly as it should be.

In the real world, in order for an event to occur, everything necessary for it to occur must have already taken place. Only when people forget this are they likely to end up justifying self-defeating behaviors with statements such as "I shoulda or woulda or coulda," all traditionally ending with "but . . ."

The obvious accurate ending for each is, of course, "But I didn't."

In fact, accurate reflection would add "I didn't because, at that particular moment, I did what I believed, under the prevailing circumstances, would work. In fact, I only questioned my behavior when it failed to achieve the gain I had anticipated."

Unfortunately, such mental confusion leads the typical client or patient, whom I will hence refer to as the consumer, to sincerely believe that he or she should have acted differently. So when I respond to such dialogues, I always start with "No, you should not have" and quickly remind them that "All conscious behavior is a product of how you think."

The progression of the dialogue is as follows: *Thinking* is the word used to describe what the brain does when it processes available information or stimuli (similar to a personal computer processing input).

The human computer (HC), your brain, like the mechanical personal computer (PC), comes with a programmed package. I believe the significant difference is this: the HC is designed to ensure the survival of the species. (I'll discuss this in more detail later). Like the PC, additional information can be added to expand the HC's performance. Unlike the PC, the HC is not only aware of its existence; it is continually modifying itself, based simply on materials it comes into contact with moment by moment. In the PC, decision making is referred to as "processing." In the HC, we generally refer to it as "thinking."

Both PC and HC are limited by the quality of information they are provided. The HC's potential, however, is further complicated by unsolicited input such as morality and ethics. So whereas basic programming is simply wired to achieve/ensure survival, as societies and cultures have evolved, the human evolution has been required to incorporate these ethics and moral factors into the game plan. Survival instincts must now incorporate new data associated with factors provided by the dominant social structure, and this information must be learned. It is not a part of that data the human genome has been hot-wired with from birth. (The PC does not have to contend with and is therefore not confused by such factors.) The fact is much of the new data is not specific to the individual environment. Many are able to survive without it. Humans, in fact, assimilate or discard/ignore information in ratio to their individual perception of how this new data has been demonstrated to positively versus negatively impact their individual lives. That is, the amount of pain or discomfort an individual is willing to endure, in most cases, may be associated to the level of gain attained or expected. Acceptable pain tends to correlate with anticipated gain. All human behaviors, therefore, have as their initial goal some positive benefit and, therefore, make perfectly good sense to the person doing/engaged in the behavior.

For example, what motivates a masochist to endure, in fact seek, pain? To the casual observer, it makes no sense, but when questioning or attempting to understand consumer behaviors to establish a therapeutic relationship, all one truly needs to understand is that the behavior makes perfect sense to the masochist. If the individual consumer is able/willing to accept this simple fact, they will rarely find themselves unnecessarily upset about the actions of others. They will find themselves more capable of utilizing personal time and energy to explore more personally satisfying ways to recognize how their actions affect not only themselves but also other significant people in their lives. With this thought in mind, one will rarely find him/herself unduly upset over the behaviors of others.

One of the more often repeated clichés, "Thinking the same thoughts and expecting that some aspect of your life will change," is often used by members of various helping professions to describe consumer behaviors that, to the observer, may border on "insanity." I sincerely hope this reading will help you make sense of the nonsense of such rhetoric.

CHAPTER FIVE

Making Sense of Your World

As previously stated, people don't engage in behaviors that, to them, do not make sense.

Again, things we do often make little or no sense to those observing, but at the moment, they always appear to make sense to the person engaged in the behavior.

For example, burglars who get caught on numerous occasions may ask themselves, "how could I be so stupid?" Are they truly suggesting that they are stupid? Of course not; they are merely pointing out how unfortunate it was that they were apprehended.

I have worked in the helping profession for over twenty-five years. During this time, I have never had a mentally ill person or substance abuser say his or her intent was to become mentally ill or chemically dependent. I have never heard a gambler say their intent was to lose their money or emotionally harm others close to them. After several years of abstinence and repairing the damage done by the last failed attempt to control their compulsion, they find themselves succumbing to that voice that whispers, "How about a quick half an hour at the casino before you head home?" How hours later, broke and disgusted, they find themselves banging their heads against the wall admonishing themselves, "How could I be so stupid?"

They all suggest, "It just seemed to happen," and this appears to be the case with most, if not all, habitual/compulsion-driven behaviors. They just seem to happen.

What about the boxer who gets in the ring every other week and gets beaten black-and-blue . . . just to pay the rent? Not knowing the motive, does it make sense to the casual observer? Of course not!

How does the professional community address the issues resulting from habitual behaviors? Usually by assigning labels, e.g., "addict."

You see, it's a characterological thing. That's just what addicts do!

Over the years, the helping profession has gone to great lengths to mystify and thereby strengthen the mystique associated with the illnesses that fall in the category of addictive behaviors and are most commonly assigned to issues associated with chemical dependence. This has traditionally been accomplished with lengthy rhetoric and neologisms that have done little more than reinforce long-standing concepts, even though many no longer meet the test of scrutiny. For example, in a survey I regularly perform at seminars or during classes, I randomly select participants and ask them to describe the conditions that result from a disease. Consistently, the overwhelming majority conclude it is "a condition that is both contracted and transmittable." small percentage will describe it as a state of personal discomfort, and an even smaller percent will be willing to acknowledge they did not know.

Don't Rock the Boat

For many of us, questioning the paradigms related to disease and addiction requires a herculean effort. Many find it difficult to "create waves" when the accepted mantra is to "just go along," "don't rock the boat." To this day, I must consciously challenge myself not to just accept or go along, remain stoic in the belief that I should stick to those principles I believe in and continue to place faith in simple concepts I understand and have found to work for me. They are the following:

* People engage in compulsive-type behaviors (which happen to include abusive use of alcohol and other drugs) because the behavior, whatever it may be, serves some functional purpose for them, e.g., for the individual, it works!

   To the person indulging in the behavior, it makes perfect sense.

   The sometimes- or often-negative results just don't seem to make sense at all and are therefore usually labeled as "nonsense." (If it made sense, it would not be perceived as a problem.)

* Effective counseling or self-help programs/groups enable participants to make sense of what they usually interpret as nonsense and requires accurate information, information the consumer usually has not had access to.

   Effective counseling provides the individual with the accurate information they need to develop solutions to the challenges that exist in their world. In short, accurate information and practice will enable the consumers you counsel to counsel him or herself more effectively in the future.

* Once again, events of daily living, which we are motivated to address, are merely challenges. They only take on the magnitude associated to the word *problem* when circumstances are perceived as either undesirable or unattainable.

* Accurate information is the base upon which solutions are formed and provides the motivation for one to engage in the problem-solving process.

CHAPTER SIX

A Language That Makes Sense

Oral communication is one of the most misunderstood forms of art, mostly because people assume they are competent in its use. For this reason, these same people become terribly distraught when their messages are not understood the way they want or need them to be understood. In daily dialogue, people find themselves consistently saying what they don't mean, meaning what they don't say and becoming upset when their message is not responded to as they intended. Such is the nonsense that exists in our daily attempts at communication.

Many years ago, I attended a lecture and first heard these words: "I'm sure you think you understood what I said, but what you don't understand is what you think you heard is not what I meant." Through the years, I have found this to represent the typical miscommunication model, and I regularly use it in my lectures to explain the communication process. It helps to clear up any confusion you, the listener or reader, may have as to what constitutes effective communication.

At the most elemental level, we are all aware that the ability to simply draw a picture does not make one an artist; special skills, vision, and talent turn a drawing into art. The ability to articulate a language does not qualify one as a communicator. Like an artist, a communicator uses his media to assist others in seeing and understanding the world as he sees or understands it, and this ability turns words into an art form. So the ability to communicate with oneself effectively is an art form. Art forms can be learned; you need only give yourself a good enough reason to make the effort.

My sincere hope is that each reader will notice that the focus of this text is on the communication/language-specific skills required to effectively engage in dialogue with yourself and others. It is anticipated that each reader will use the concepts discussed to help identify self-talk, which impedes their ability to attain and sustain their most personally desired emotional goals. By definition, such conversations can be labeled as self-defeating, and the obvious goal of self-counseling would be to acquire methods for restructuring these dialogues in ways that will assist them to better achieve their personal and most desired emotional goals.

The available self-help modules titled "Making Sense of the Nonsense" are designed to assist consumers in developing those skills that will help them to identify and more effectively cope with those elements of their personal life that trigger self-defeating emotional or behavioral responses. As a result of completing the self-help modules connected with this text, it is anticipated that the individual reader/consumer will be able to identify those emotional responses associated with specific life events that are problematic.

Finally, I sincerely hope each reader will find him or herself motivated to investigate the other resources offered by the CSSHC that may assist them to develop techniques that will assist in developing new responses that will achieve problem/conflict resolution to the daily stressors they will surely be confronted with in the future.

A Common Language

In arrogance assumed most specifically by speakers of the English language, it is assumed that only those peoples of a savage or of an unenlightened nature are incapable of understanding dialogues conducted in this tongue. Since American English (probably the most ravaged of all the languages) is, in fact, a very imprecise medium, and since its speakers are required to use this imprecise tool to communicate, not only with others, but more importantly, with themselves, the resulting confusion is fairly predictable.

Many years ago, I concluded that mental health professionals are as guilty of faulty or flawed communication as any of those persons they are committed to provide assistance to. Additionally, they often sabotage their altruistic efforts by attempting to motivate consumers to change their physical or emotional responses to those worldly events that generate them without changing the way they think about the events to which they are responding.

Without going into the details of why, many of my colleagues and I have for years suggested that this is a specific form of lunacy. Lunacy, being described as "people's attempts to feel or behave differently while thinking the same thoughts that generated the behavior or emotions they are trying to change." We then wonder why are there so many people in general and consumers specifically who are in a state of confusion and wondering why.

The major portion of my counseling career has been spent in efforts to help myself and others make sense of the nonsense of such rhetoric. As previously stated, my initial efforts were based upon tested and accepted cognitive/behavior theories. My efforts here are to communicate the ideas and concepts of these theories in a dialogue I hope will be more easily internalized by the average consumer.

Since most of the information being presented will be related to theories that are cognitively based. Let's start by clarifying the terms generally associated with the term *cognition*. They are *cognitive, cognitive distortion, sense*, and *nonsense.*

Webster's New Twentieth Century Dictionary defines *cognitive* as "[one's] ability to know, perceive, be aware," e.g., make sense of the world or environment they are relegated to live in.

Life and the individual events associated with living make sense if one either understands it or believes they are benefiting from it. Additionally, such events in life are mutually exclusive. That is, if one understands a situation or event, they may accept "the sense of it," though they may not necessarily benefit from it. On the other hand, if one is benefiting from the same situation, they may not necessarily feel a need to understand why. If one neither understands nor benefits from an event or situation, they will likely view it as nonsense.

Webster's definition of *cognitive distortion* is "to twist out of its original shape; to misrepresent [intentional or not]." It (cognitive distortion) is a misrepresentation of what one knows, either consciously or unconsciously. Cognitive distortions are classic forms of self-deceit or nonsense.

To fully understand the concept of cognitive distortion, one must first acknowledge some basics. Let's begin with perception. It is generally accepted that to establish perception, you must first be exposed to a stimulus, e.g., encounter a situation (event). In some manner, the event must impact on you as an individual. You must, in some way, become aware that something (the event) has taken place. We experience this awareness through our senses. That is, we must see it, hear it, touch it, smell it, taste it. With varying degrees of intensity, we experience these sensations as positive (good feelings), negative (pain or dis-ease), or neutral. The impact is generally dependent on the manner in which the event impacts on the individual's potential to survive.

Though it may seem simplistic, as far as I am able to determine, this is the range of human feelings and emotions.

However, on close examination, such simple concepts may become complicated.

For instance, does what your eyes see accurately represent the real world?

Well . . . not exactly.

Physiologically, what your eyes see are reflections of light beams that the brain compiles into a construct and stores for future reference and, when called upon, will play back in HD Blu-ray on the wide screen of your mind. In our simplicity, we simply perceive it as a picture. Now you're probably thinking, "Like a videotape or camera?"

Well . . . no! Not nearly that simplistic.

Remember, the brain, as we know or perceive it, has few, if any, limitations. Without manipulation, a camera can only show you what exists or is objective reality.

The brain has no such limitations. It has been noted (Maultsby 1976) that the brain "can take what you know to exist or see and, based upon your personal hopes, dreams, fears or nightmares, subjectively distort the reality." For this reason, to experience mental and emotional health, our subjective views of the world or our truths must conform to the objective realities/facts of our daily life. This is a basic requirement for eliminating emotional confusion. It represents the foundation of the most popularly accepted cognitively based theories. This insight should strengthen your ability to make sense of the nonsense that may exist in your world. So what do we know about truth?

Truth feels good. So, when our personal truths come into conflict with the realities/facts associated with our life circumstances, we often find ourselves resorting to that other uniquely human trait rationalization. Yes! We humans are the only animal on the planet with the unique ability to rationalize. e.g feel good in circumstances we most certainly should not feel good in. Facts, on the other hand, are cold and not subject to rationalization, regardless of the level of discomfort they may generate, Facts simply exist and emotionally healthy people learn to adapt and cope with them. Sort of like having big feet, you accept they're going to be there, for a long time.

CHAPTER SEVEN

More About Feelin' Good

I make a point here to emphasize the distinct difference between "feeling" and "feelin' good." Where "feeling" is generally associated with a tactile experience, the colloquial understanding of "feelin'" is akin to how one is experiencing the emotional aspects of their world. For instance, "feelin'" happy. Though most consumers seeking help from professionals haven't the slightest idea what it will take to make them happy, they are, nonetheless, actively engaged in pursuing that "feelin'" associated with happiness.

The fact is very few of those persons seeking happiness know a proven, effective technique for achieving it.

Ask a friend to define *happiness.*

I assure you, the most commonly accepted definition will allude to "feelin' good." Many, therefore, have resorted to alcohol and other drugs (AOD) as the solution.

Why?

Because they work!

One thing we have all learned since childhood is that there is a pill or potion that will temporarily relieve physical or emotional discomfort, and the learned form of thinking, which suggests that the realities of one's world are going to change simply because they feel better, is a prime contributor being reinforced through media resources daily, and the insanity associated to the addicted mind is surely a product of the way we have been programmed to process our world. Let's take a brief look at the origin of this programming.

Where the natural drive is to accomplish behaviors that provide a personal good feelin' as a payoff, the societal mandate is to accomplish behaviors that are rewarding to others, and this is generally referred to as *doin' good.* Where society demands that you ought to do good is reinforced by good feelin's, the want/desire to feel good does not in and of itself manifests as good deeds/doin' good. In fact, where doin' good may reinforce the desire to perform more good deeds in hope of that good feelin' payoff, feelin' good, it appears, leads to a desire to simply feel even better, and this prepares us to take a look at how AOD /Compulsion-driven behaviors may currently be impacting your life.

Did you ever feel like you needed something outside of yourself just to kinda help you

        loosen up so you could have a little fun?   _____
        communicate socially/get your game on?   _____
        just plain relax?   _____
        cope with normal daily situations?   _____
        get your day started?   _____

A yes response to any one of the above is a sign that you are probably, at least, psychologically dependent on something outside of yourself for your sense of well-being, which is the first step toward addictive-type behaviors that include chemical/drug dependence.

Remember this: No person awakes one morning and decides that they are going to wreck their life or the lives of others who are close to them by succumbing to some form of addictive behavior. Such events are generally the accidental result of people attempting to find happiness or release or relief through resources outside of themselves.

In the case of drugs or alcohol, it may be described as people attempting to medicate or drink rather than think themselves into a preferred emotional/feeling state, which is equivalent to the state most sought through other forms of self-defeating behaviors that have been labeled "addictions."

Here's the good news.

As long as you have your normally functioning brain, you don't have to be dependent on forces outside of yourself or chemicals to experience good feelin's or to attain a sense of well-being. You can learn to experience the feelin'/emotions you want/desire to feel, at will, through the use of simple common sense skills, and you can accomplish this without engaging in potentially addictive/self-destructive behaviors or the use of drugs. My personal workbook series Making Sense of the Nonsense and most other cognitively oriented theories have been designed to teach the skills necessary to accomplish cognitive/behavioral change.

CHAPTER EIGHT

Understanding Feelings

Over the years, we have come to understand that feelings fall generally into two categories: physical and emotional.

Physical feelings are simple to understand. You touch hot stove, you get burned (pain). Stick finger with needle? It hurts (pain). A fur coat in cold weather feels warm (good). To have someone remove a two-hundred-pound rock from your chest feels good.

Emotional feelings (feelin's), on the other hand, are generally more complicated to understand.

Though feelin's are often presented as "easy as ABC," the actual process through which we experience an emotional feelin' is more complicated and, therefore, more often misinterpreted or misunderstood. So let's take a look at them.

The ABCs of Emotional Feelin's

In counseling, patrons often ask this:

(Q) Are emotions really as simple as ABC?
(A) Yes! But simple does not necessarily equate to easy.

Therefore, when confronted with what appears to be a complicated emotional dilemma, clients/patrons will often think to themselves, *I'm fairly intelligent. I studied psychology. If my emotions were really so simple, I certainly would have figured them out by now.*

But the fact is they often haven't figured them out.

Therefore, they will normally want to reject the simplicity of the ABC model: it's simply not mind-boggling enough. They prefer to believe that their emotions are uncontrollable and incomprehensibly complex, and this frees them from responsibility for any subsequent actions. To help patients and clients free themselves from such nonsense, the professional must assist the individual patron to understand why they missed discovering their emotional ABCs, on their own, in the first place, and this presents an ideal opportunity for the therapist/clinician to point out that at the moment in question, their thinking was not sufficiently or correctly focused.

When thinking about the causes of emotions, people rarely look at their thoughts; the immediate tendency is to focus on the external world: the he, she, and it that appear to be causing their emotions.

Why?

Maybe because at that moment, their emotions were so intensely distracting, or possibly because accepting that the emotions being experienced were a product of their thinking and that thinking is the one aspect of our lives that we do, in fact, have control over carries with it too much responsibility. You see, acknowledging/accepting the idea that one controls his or her emotions is extremely empowering, and once the individual is able to accept this concept, they can no longer blame the he's, she's, and it's of the world for (their feelin's) making them feel anything emotionally. It also eliminates the best emotional cop-out existing: "the devil made me do it." Accepting this kind of control, the individual becomes too sophisticated to continue playing these kinds of emotional games on themselves.

Regardless of the reason, when people focus primarily on the external world to explain their emotions, they keep themselves emotionally naive. But once they learn and accept the following, they are able to free themselves to feel the emotions they want to feel when they want to feel them.

Though most human emotions are often defined as "simple as ABC," contrary to accepted ABC teachings, the initial exposure is not linear.

Let's do a quick review of the classic ABC process.

The classic ABC process describes A as the "antecedent" or the event/circumstance to which one has been exposed. B is described as the belief system one has developed about the event at A, which results in a "behavior" one executes as a result of this exposure and is represented at C as a "consequence" of that behavior.

The common sense concept of the ABC process suggests that the initial exposure is, in fact, an ACB response set (an event at A that results in an affect/emotion at C—positive, negative, neutral) that is stored and thereafter accessed as a product of the belief system established relevant to the event. Once this correlation has been established, the process then takes on the ABC format/ response set which, if repeated over time, will eventually result in a more simplistic AC response, which is generally acknowledged as a habit.

For example, pain may be the result of touching a pinpoint (in fact) or through exposure to information (vicarious). Until experienced in one form or another, the physical or emotional impact of pain cannot be anticipated. Once this exposure has occurred, future responses both physical or emotional can thereafter be mediated, thus ABC. A belief system is now established, which, in future situations, may offer the option to avoid the pain associated with touching the pinpoint.

Once again, an initial encounter will flow something like this:

A. An event takes place in your life.
B. It impacts your life in a positive, negative, or neutral manner, and that encounter is stored in your computer bank (HC) as such.

C. Future behavioral or emotional responses will be predicated on this stored information.

Your initial ACB response set has now become an ABC response set.

A. Your perceptions: How/what you notice about your world impacts on one or more of your five senses
plus
B. Your sincere (positive, negative, or neutral) thoughts about your perceptions
plus
C. Your (positive, negative, or neutral) gut or emotional feelings triggered by your memory/stored thoughts (B) relevant to this event

Simple emotional ignorance is not the only reason most people initially resist learning their emotional ABCs. There are at least two other reasons.

First, most people have tried (more than once) and failed to change their emotional feelings about specific situations. They then misinterpret this as proof that they had no control over their emotions in the first place.

Second, according to Maultsby (1976), "People don't always experience their emotions in a logical ABC sequence." As previously discussed, people rarely perceive at A and think at B before they act or experience an emotional feeling at C.

What most often happens is people perceive at A and habitually/instantly react with a behavior or an emotional feelin' at C without having had time to think anything. They see no problem with the reaction simply because it was emotional, and remember, emotions just happen; we are not responsible for emotions, especially those that do not feel good.

Points to Remember

It is anticipated that you will read this short text more than once, so do not attempt to analyze the material word for word. You will find the material most useful if you simply read through it several times—until it makes sense or you are able to discuss the material with someone who may assist you. If you are a student, see your counselor; if you are a therapist, see your workshop leader or discuss with a fellow professional.

This material is presented to help you to help yourself and, hopefully, eventually help others to understand themselves and to change aspects of their lives they may find problematic. It is expected that you will eventually pass this material on, but before you do, take a few moments and answer the following questions:

1. Does any part of what I have read apply to me?
   _____ (Yes) _____ (No)
2. Have I ever acted on any of the insights I have just read about? ___ (Yes) _____ (No)
   a. If you answered yes to question no. 2, give a specific example of how you acted on those insights. _____
   _____
   b. Briefly describe the results of acting on those insights.
   _____ _____
   _____
3. In what future situations could you apply those insights?
   _____ _____
   _____

Be sure to go over your insights with someone you trust and feel comfortable with.

CHAPTER NINE

Clearing-up Mental Confusion

How Can This Information Help an Individual in Recovery?

One of the most common reasons people in recovery relapse (return to previously identified problem behavior) is that they confuse wanting to engage in an old behavior such drinking or drug use with craving that behavior.

Note: Although alcohol is the example used here, the general principles discussed apply to all compulsion-driven behaviors. Once people suffering from such behaviors understand the mechanisms that control craving, wanting, desiring, and needing, they free themselves to feel, emotionally, the way they want to feel without resorting to problem behaviors such as the abusive use of alcohol or other addictive drugs. In order to accomplish this, it is important that you become familiar with the terms most associated with the relapse process.

Primary versus Secondary Cravings

Primary cravings are unavoidable and intense urges to participate in specific behaviors or to ingest an addictive drug. These urges occur when the brain neurochemistry is insufficient to maintain a normal state of calm or homeostasis. (See Blum et al.)

In the case of drug addiction, primary cravings occur only in the secondary stage. The greater the depletion of normal neurochemicals or loss of the drug, the more severe and powerful the primary cravings become until (in the case of chemical dependency) one of the following three things occur:

* Enough of the addictive drug is ingested to supplement the absence of the natural neurochemicals and thus stop the craving and restore a drug-induced sense of well-being or physiologic homeostasis.
* The chemically dependent individual opts to go through withdrawal without a substitute drug (cold turkey).
* The consumer/patient receives medical detoxification and reestablishes a healthy physiologic balance (homeostasis) naturally (without drugs).

With this information at hand, you must wonder why most alcoholics do choose more alcohol.

The answer, though frightening, is really very simple. To get medically detoxified requires the time, effort, and the inconvenience of going to the hospital or possibly jail. Unfortunately, until the individual suffering from chemical dependency is absolutely helpless, they have access to their drug of choice much quicker and with fewer problems than that required to gain access to a hospital or jail.

Going cold turkey is a quick means of detoxification, but it is also the most frightening, painful, and dangerous means of getting clean or sober. Up to 25 percent of alcoholics who go cold turkey die in the process. It is, therefore, understandable that most sobering-up alcoholics choose more alcohol.

Secondary Cravings

Though secondary cravings feel similar to primary cravings, the similarity ends with the feeling. Where primary cravings are the body's physical cry for help, secondary cravings are merely the minds' habitual responses to the use of alcohol or other drugs (AOD) in situations associated with past circumstances, where a perceived or real benefit was derived from its use.

It is important here to emphasize that rarely, if ever, do habitual responses develop to behaviors that serve no purpose. In short, the drinking or drug-using behavior most probably served a definite need when it was first developed.

For example, take a problem drinker who habitually drinks in bars to ease his shyness and guilt about seeking companionship. He finds that one or two shots of his favorite nerve booster, a central nervous system depressant (CNSD), e.g., alcohol, helps to numb the guilt associated with this behavior and, in fact, has enabled him to overcome his shyness long enough to carry on a conversation and to make a date or learn and join in the latest "line dance".

And let's assume that the following week he was able, with the help of two or three shots, to accomplish the same task. The message is "alcohol works." The following morning, he is still shy, but he has made opposite-sex contact. He may honestly not want to drink anymore. But next weekend, the memory is still there that it worked, and the probability is he will try again, and if it continues to work (suppress his shyness thus enabling him to communicate), this cue will trigger a secondary craving for alcoholic drinks.

Unfortunately, traditional alcoholic treatment programs rarely teach alcoholics the difference between secondary cravings (which are generally perceived as harmless) and the early stage of their more dangerous old primary cravings. Consequently, when people in recovery experience secondary cravings, they are often confused, afraid, and often, quite disgusted with themselves.

They were probably convinced that their last treatment or stay in jail had cured them. They quickly forgot the nature of their illness and easily convinced themselves that treatment didn't really work. In many cases, many will simply give up and return to their previous destructive behaviors, even though it was not their intent to do so.

Giving up is largely a product of a flawed belief system that suggests that being in recovery means never craving alcohol or other drugs again. In the alcohol-free environment of a treatment facility or program, the absence of an environment to trigger the urges to use or to drink provides little to no stimulus to drink, and the craving response is generally mild or nonexistent/extinct. It, therefore, makes sense that under such conditions most will believe, "I've been cured" and leave their treatment programs sincerely expecting never again to experience the craving response again. This is, of course, akin to never again experiencing or recalling your favorite pet or first girlfriend. Try that and see how well it works!

Unfortunately, therapists and counselors often allow these naive expectations to develop. Regardless, it doesn't change the facts of your life or situation. In the real world of addiction or compulsion-driven behaviors, one quickly comes face-to-face with those cues that have historically triggered their craving responses—restaurants, bars, parties, intense negative emotional states, etc.—and predictably, these cues will trigger secondary craving responses.

In the resulting confusion, the individual being driven by a compulsion will quickly forget the nature/permanence of their illness and think, "Damn! I've just been fooling myself. I thought I was cured. After all the crap I've been through with drugs, etc., and trying to get well, here I am wanting to use/subjecting myself to the same stuff all over again. I really must be as low as everyone said I was! I'm no better than that bum on the corner I used to hold in such low esteem. How could I have sunk to this depth?"

Such self-denigrating thoughts are bound to trigger strong negative emotions. These negative emotions, combined with secondary cravings, will tend to intensify the total level of discomfort. The resulting secondary cravings then appear more like the potentially dangerous primary cravings.

At this point, the person in recovery often panics and convinces him/herself that only their drug of choice can help them. They've just got to have a drink, etc.

Sincere thoughts such as "need to have" or "got to have" are the strongest human motivators for immediate action. Such uninformed and confused thinking will predictably result in a return to addictive behavior, i.e., drinking or using other drugs. The user will quickly feel relief and conclude, "Well, I may as well go on and enjoy myself until I have to go in for treatment again. Maybe next time, I'll get a big-enough dose of treatment to really cure me."

To assist those in recovery to avoid such self-defeating ends, it is important that they learn the following relatively objective way to recognize and separate wishes and wants and primary craving and secondary cravings.

Wishing and Wanting

Wishing and wanting are childhood constructs that result in the development of thinking processes that often manifests in adulthood as mystical thinking. Between the approximate ages of two and six, children tend to believe that by simply wishing for or wanting something, it ought to happen. Past this age range or at least by adulthood, it is assumed that we will develop a level of cognition or awareness that enables us to realize that in a nonmystical or nonmagical world, things or events only happen when all the things necessary to make them happen have, in fact, occurred.

By adulthood, through normal cognitive development, we realize that wishes and wants are merely mental constructs of something we desire. This desire is usually predicated on the belief that by having it, our lives would be more complete, if we were to get what we want or wish for, simply because we want or wish for it. See the nonsense of this form of thinking? In fact, "because wishes and wants are merely mental constructs/thoughts, they exist only in [the] mind," and because, by now you realize that you and you alone control your mind, which controls your belief system, which determines your perceptions of your world, it is likely that you may now be willing to accept that you can change your thoughts and perceptions at will. Now, since wishing equates to magical thinking, unless you are a magician, it shouldn't be too difficult to acknowledge that your wishes are generally a construct of a desire for an event that cannot or probably will not happen without significant effort from you. For example, you may wish to have a lot of money. Wants, on the other hand, usually represent desires or events that could happen if all the necessary things to make them happen do, in fact, happen. The key here is the work associated with doing all the necessary things. That is, having not accomplished all the required tasks to ensure an event happening, an individual may attempt to delude themselves with self-statements such as "There's no good reason for this happening to me" or with pseudoquestions such as "Why is this happening?" or more specifically, "Why is this happening to me?" that suggests there is no reason or that this, in fact, should not be happening. This is obvious cognitive distortion, and it is obvious cognitive distortion because they never answer these forms of question. Why? Because they are not truly questions. They are simple statements of the belief that "this should not be happening to me!"

People obsessed with wanting things are generally unwilling or unable to do all the things necessary to make the desired events happen, and that is the answer to their why question. They are usually unmotivated or unwilling to engage in the type of sustained activity required to achieve their wants. Circumstances are often so overwhelming, the individual, so as not to have to admit defeat, will deny ever having had the desire or want, for example, the thought "I want to be a doctor."

Acknowledging all the steps necessary to accomplish this goal and not believing you have access to the tools might be sufficient enough to discourage you from accepting it as an achievable goal. The result could easily be giving up on the desire by labeling it as inaccessible.

Believing you are unable to make an event happen will often result in a refusal to engage in those activities necessary to make it happen.

Hopes and Desires

Though writers of dictionaries may not agree with all that follows, I ask that you keep in mind that they were not in the business of helping people and certainly not of treating people suffering from mental illnesses or substance abuse. Additionally, their goal was to define and not necessarily to help people to communicate more precisely or efficiently.

Hopes and desires are linear (ABC type) constructs. They consist of perceived events/objects at A (getting a skateboard for Christmas), ideas of want at B (all the fun to be had skateboarding), plus positive goal-directed urges at C (behaviors he will have to exhibit to get the desired/wanted objects at A.

Unlike wishes and wants, hopes pleasantly motivate you . . . (to engage in sustained goal-directed actions/activity).

CHAPTER TEN

The Common Sense Perspective of Needs

Maslow's hierarchy has taught us that there are objective human needs. Objective meaning that these needs exist outside or independently of our basic human wants, desires, or demands. To stay alive, we need food, water, and shelter (i.e., protection from life-threatening events. (It is also accepted that the human animal needs love/nurturing).

To be happy, sad, or calm, healthy people need (i.e. must have) happy, sad, or calm beliefs and attitudes. These are neurologic and psychophysiologic facts. They exist whether or not people know about them, believe them, or choose to deny them. Common sense forces us to focus on our objective needs. On the other hand, a subjective need exists in the mind of the believer. It consists of a strong desire to have something, plus a self-imposed personal punishment for not getting it.

For example, many of us believe that to feel satisfied with ourselves, we need the love or approval of certain other people. In fact, they don't need that love or approval; they just want it so much, they are (unconsciously) willing to make themselves miserable (i.e. punish themselves) when they believe they are not getting it.

What motivates people to such self-destructive behavior? Primarily fear. Fear of the miserable feelings they self-generate to punish themselves for not being deserving of the love or approval they wish for or want.

Fortunately, the need for love or approval is subjective. It exists only in the individual mind, and by merely changing one's mind, one can eliminate self-defeating beliefs and the conflicts they cause.

The nature of the addictive mind suggests it must have the object of its addiction (drugs, alcohol, gambling, sex) to feel emotionally better. In fact, it is merely seeking the feeling or lack of feeling ascribed to indulgence in the addictive agent, and the addict is willing to punish himself, self-defeatingly, by pointing out how miserable he/she will feel if they don't get their drug. This justifies engaging in the drug use/addictive behavior. Having engaged in their addictive agent/behavior, they get relief (feel better) and delude themselves by concluding that their relief proved they needed the drug to feel better.

Because subjective needs exist only in the mind of the believer, those dependent of AOD always have at least two means of increasing their emotional comfort: They can get what they want, or they can start to think differently and stop punishing themselves.

Often, people may fall short of getting those things they want. The good news is they can always change their minds.

To avoid mental confusion, people suffering from addictions need to remember the nature of their disease and, when confused, ask themselves, "Who's in control and of what?"

Summary

1. Wishes and wants for AOD are merely perceptions plus ideas of desires existing only in the human mind. By acknowledging this, the problem drinker or addict can instantly start or stop wishing for or wanting the subject of his or her addiction. They merely have to start to think differently about the object in question.

2. Hopes and desires for AOD are ABC-type emotions. They consist of perceptions, ideas of wants, plus positive emotive urges to get what is wanted. Hopes and desires can usually be stopped or started as quickly and in the same way as any other emotion, i.e., by a change in thoughts followed by actions designed to better get the individual needs met.

3. Primary cravings are unavoidable chemically induced states of physical distress. They are caused by depriving the body of those outside agents, i.e., AOD, which have supplemented the body's natural neurochemistry and now assists in the maintenance of its normal homeostasis.

   Primary alcoholic cravings can be both painful and life threatening. Treatment is most appropriately accomplished through medical detoxification. Addicts, in general, can stop primary cravings temporarily by engaging in the object of their addiction. They can stop permanently by cessation (cold turkey) or by seeking professional assistance and treatment.

4. Secondary cravings are learned types of habitual emotional reactions to situations or memories associated with repeated past behaviors that are now identified as problematic.

   For example, secondary cravings for alcohol are really positive memories associated with alcohol consumption that result in habitual desires for alcohol. That is why they occur involuntarily on cue even though the problem drinker doesn't want to drink alcohol anymore. Because the person no longer wants to drink, those formerly pleasant urges for a drink now result in unpleasant emotions, but they are not necessarily harmful or overpowering. That's why they can be started or stopped in the same way as any other habitual emotional reaction. As with all habits, to stop the drinking response to alcoholic cravings, the sober problem drinker must confront the belief system/memory that is generating the cravings.

To complete this summary without at least a brief reference to Anger, Stress and Conflict resolution would make the entire work appear without purpose. This short work has hopeful assisted you to understand that anger and stress are personal emotional responses to the events occurring in your world. By now it is expected that the individual reader is aware that they alone are responsible for the emotional feelings they expedience, in response to the events of life. It is anticipated that you understand that emotional responses are merely adaptive responses and when they are no longer self-serving they can be changed or discarded. It is also anticipated that you understand that in order to effect this change, the individual must develop a new way of describing the events and circumstances of their life accurately. If you've read this far, I assume you are now able to engage in a more personally satisfying Self Talk. You are now aware of the important role self talk plays and capable of engaging yourself in a more personally satisfying dialog about events of your life.

POINT OF EMPHASIS

Regardless of how much sense an idea may appear to make to you, if you are not thoroughly convinced that it is in your best interest to adopt it, don't. You are only motivated to put ideas tto work, when you are convinced that they will work for you. If you are not willing to accept an idea and attempt to adopt it into your life, you'll just end up continuing to execute your old behaviors and thinking. Of course, you could always point out to yourself that though it probably want make you any worse off, it certainly won't be helping you either.

Remember, all re-education takes time and practice. Don't demand perfection, just commit to an effort each day and you can expect steady progress toward your preferred emotional goals.

Now you may ask yourself.

Can I pretend to work on my problems, when in fact, I'm actually avoiding them?"

And the answer is??? A resounding. YES! These are the kind of emotional games highly motivated humans use to trick themselves into believing they are feeling better, without thinking better and in such cases, since they will be thinking the same way, they will also be reacting in thier usual ways and contributhng to their mental confusion, by asking themselves, Why? Then continuing to add to their confusion by not answering the question [because no true question was ever asked] and then perpetuating the ruse that there was or is any good or reasonable reason for things being as they are. Such is the lunacy associated with the games we play in our efforts to establish communication with ourselves and others. At this point,I'dlike to emphasize that [no one can stop people from playing games on themnselves]. People who play games with their efforts at self counseling would play the same games if they were paying for professional therapy or counseling. [No counselor or therapist has ever been able to prevent a determined/highly-motivated consumer from playing games on him or herself]. Such people are generally hindered by other long standing emotional problems. They are unable to control their daily lives and are therefore likely candidates for professional intervention.

When you are able to imagine yourself doing behaviors and thinking thoughts that consistently produce those behaviors, you will learn that your mistakes will rarely hurt you or anyone else; you will become capable of correcting your mistakes quickly and without fear, guilt or shame; you will enhance your potential for feeling and doing exactly what you want to do about your next real life experience or problem; you will reduce the potential that your will experience the same problem behavior again; you will find yourself capable of experiencing the feelings and feelin's you most desire, without resorting to the use of alcohol, drugs or other compulsion-driven behaviors.

Remember Emotional success, like other successes, is a product of practice and those who practice most diligently are generally most successful. Like luck, success in most endeavors tends to run in direct ratio to skill. Persons unwilling to put forth effort are unlikely candidates for self-help counseling formats and unfortunately, for such persons, no form of counseling is likely to be effective.

Question

Do You Really Have to Be so Precise in Your Dialogues with Yourself?

NO! But people attempting to cope with problem behaviors tend to desire rapid resolution and in such cases, preciseness is essential. For instance: The sincere thought "I really want it" (but meaning "I hope for or desire it") is probably the single most popular self-motivating idea people have, and the sincere thought "I've got to have it" is probably the single most powerful self-defeating idea people have. (How can you not respond to a desire to attain something you've "just got to have"? I mean, you're going to die without it, right?

When people believe they can't get the things they really want or "just have to have," they begin to believe life is not worth living. Such logic is probably the single most important reason there are revolutionaries ("Give me liberty, or give me death"), martyrs, and terrorists. In a moderately intense form, the belief "I've just got to, but I can't" is the most common cause of simple depression in everyday life. Trying to control such depressions with alcohol or other drugs is a common reason people make themselves dependent on drugs for relief.

CHAPTER ELEVEN

Compulsion-Driven Behaviors/ The Nature of Addiction

Alcohol and drug dependency is defined as "the compulsive use of mood-altering drugs." This compulsive use is characterized by a significant impairment in the individuals' ability to make common sense decisions about their life. It may individually or collectively involve physical, psychological, or social dysfunction. Individuals who are alcohol and/or drug (AOD) dependent are unable to consistently predict how much they will use or how they will behave should they make the decision to use. The resulting confusion is further fed by the numerous myths, fables, and general misinformation made available for public consumption.

The following is a list of statements about alcohol and drug dependency. Test your knowledge and understanding of the factual-base which supports each of the following statements. You'll be provided an answer sheet at the end of the session.

Test your understanding of the factual-base that supports each of the following statements. Do you agree or disagree with the statements that follow?

1. Alcohol and other drugs (AOD) have the same biochemical and physiological effect on all users.
2. AOD are addictive, and anyone who uses enough for long enough will likely develop, minimally, a psychobiological dependence.
3. Addiction is often psychological.
4. There is a well-defined addictive personality.
5. True personality is revealed when a person is intoxicated.
6. Individuals recovering from AOD often continue to be depressed, anxious, irritable, and unhappy. This is proof that the disease is caused by psychological factors.
7. Psychotherapy can help the AOD-dependent individual achieve sobriety.
8. An AOD-dependent person must want help before anything meaningful can happen.
9. Some AOD-dependent individuals can recover and return to "social use" without ill effects as long as they are able to limit their use to a specific amount.
10. AOD dependency is a single disease, and the treatment is the same for everyone.

SELF-TEST ANSWERS

1. In fact: Clearly, individual differences exist as to the level of pleasure/displeasure and sedation/excitation derived from the use of AOD.

2. In fact: Genetic susceptibility often leads to addiction. Of the U.S. population, 10 percent have the genetic background and may, therefore, be predisposed to become chemically dependent should they initiate AOD use (70 percent among Native Americans).

   Despite heavy use, only 10 percent of the soldiers returning from Vietnam who used heroin while they were there became addicted after returning to the United States.

3. In fact: Though heavy use or abuse may be a product of psychological factors alone, chemical dependence (addiction), a compulsive use in the face of definite adverse consequences, most often will have a genetic/biological predisposition.

4. In fact: Numerous studies have been unable to identify the "addictive personality." Only a family history of addiction is known to increase the incidence of addiction. "However, after addiction occurs, personality traits, such as poor self-image and poor reality testing, are often found on psychological tests."

5. In fact: AOD are known to cause disruption of brain function and to produce alterations in perception of reality and emotional responses.

6. In fact: It may take months to years for cognitive functioning to return following AOD dependency. Studies suggests that as the maturing process is often disrupted and delayed, coupled with the resulting poor self-image and poor reality testing, psychological counseling is generally required.

7. In fact: Though early support groups for anger and stress management have been found to be very helpful in the recovery process, other studies suggests that too early involvement in resolving problems may inc re se relapse potential this should be addressed with consideration for individual strengths and weaknesses.

8. In fact: Numerous counseling methods have been found to be effective in breaking through the denial system of individuals suffering from compulsion-driven behaviors. However, anyone attempting intervention must do the following:
    1. Learn about the illness
    2. Avoid making moral judgments.
    3. Be able to remain emotionally detached.
    4. If nonprofessional, seek assistance from someone who has experience in interventions.
        The lack of any of the above items (especially no. 4) may lead to an ineffective (possibly damaging) intervention and increased denial (resistance to recovery).

9. In fact: AOD-dependent individuals are never able to safely return to the use of AOD.

10. In fact: Although alcohol and other drug dependencies have a common biochemical/genetic background. They may manifest with varying expressions of severity and be evident based upon the individual's susceptibility to different chemicals.

Treatment planning must recognize the different physiological, psychological, socioeconomic, and cultural factors that may need to be addressed.

Once you've eliminated basic confusions by exposing yourself to the facts associated with the abusive use of alcohol and other drugs, you are more able to confront the nature of your baseline belief system.

Is it self-serving or self-defeating?

And now that you've answered your question . . .

INDEX

A

addiction, 13, 16, 20, 22, 29, 39, 50, 53, 58–62, 64, 66
addictive personality, 64, 66
alcohol and other addictive drugs (AOAD), 11–12, 20–21, 37–38, 52, 59–60, 62, 64–68
autistic syndrome disorders (ASDs), 21

B

Babkoff, Harvey, 15
    "Use of Stimulants to Ameliorate the Effects of Sleep Loss During Sustained Performance," 15
behaviors
    addictive/self-destructive, 29, 39, 54, 58
    compulsion-driven/habitual, 13, 22–23, 27–28, 50, 53, 62
    self-defeating, 24, 32, 39, 47, 54

C

central nervous system depressant (CNSD), 52
cessation, 61
chemical dependence. See addiction
choice, 24, 47
cognitive distortion, 34–35, 55
cognitive functioning, 67
cold turkey, 51, 61
compulsion, 7, 20, 27
coronary heart disease (CHD), 10
counseling, 30, 41
cravings
    primary, 50–52, 54, 60–61
    secondary, 50–54, 61

D

Damasio, Antonio, 12, 21
desires, 55–57, 60–61
drugs
    abuse of, 12, 21
    addictive, 11, 20, 50–51
    administration of, 12, 21

mood-altering, 62
stimulant, 13, 15, 22

E

emotional confusion, 36
emotional ignorance, 44
ethics, 25, 48

F

feelin,' 37–39, 41–42
  emotional, 41, 44
    ABC process, 43
feeling, physical, 41
feelin' good, 21, 37–38

G

genetic imbalance, 18
genetic susceptibility, 66

H

habits, 7, 43
happiness, 18, 37, 39
homeostasis, 13, 22, 50–51, 60
hopes, 56–57, 60
human computer (HC), 25

I

ice. See methamphetamine

K

Krueger, Gerald P., 15
  "Use of Stimulants to Ameliorate the Effects of Sleep Loss During Sustained Performance," 15

L

Leileilani (single mother), 15–16
lunacy, 33

M

Making Sense of the Nonsense, 32
Maslow, Abraham, 57
memory, 7, 44, 52, 61
mental illness substance abuse (MISA), 19
methamphetamine, 15–16
"Methamphetamine Effects on Cognitive Processing During Extended Wakefulness" (Weigmann, Stanny, et al.), 15
miscommunication model, 31
morality, 25, 48

N

National Institute on Alcohol Abuse and Alcoholism (NIAAA), 10, 19 needs, 57, 59–60

O

oral communication, 31

P

performance-enhancing drugs (PEDs), 16
personal computer (PC), 25, 48

R

relapse, 50, 67
replacement behavior, 8

S

self-image, 66–67
self-talk, 32
Stanny, Robert R., 15
  "Methamphetamine Effects on Cognitive Processing During Extended Wakefulness," 15
stressors, 18

T

thinking, 12, 21, 25, 42, 48, 54–55
tranquilizers, 13, 22

W

wanting, 50, 54, 56, 60
wants, 54–57, 60
Weigmann, Douglas A.
  "Methamphetamine Effects on Cognitive Processing During Extended Wakefulness," 15
wishing, 54–55, 60

www.ingramcontent.com/pod-product-compliance
Lightning Source LLC
Chambersburg PA
CBHW030010190526
45157CB00014B/2092